The Diabetes Code

Natural Ways to Reverse Type 2 Diabetes

Harmony Royce

Copyright © 2024 Harmony Royce

All rights reserved.

DEDICATION

This book is dedicated to everyone who bravely, resolutely, and determinedly faces the obstacles posed by diabetes. I hope the anecdotes in these pages provide you with motivation and that you learn useful techniques to help you on your path to improved health. For those on similar pathways, your dedication to self-care and your unflinching attitude in the face of hardship serve as a light of hope. Let's work together to create a day when diabetes is recognized, treated, and eventually cured.

CONTENTS

Disclaimer..8
ACKNOWLEDGMENTS... 1
CHAPTER 1... 1
The Big Lie About Type 2 Diabetes 1.. 1

1.1: The Myth - The Reason We Believe Type 2 Diabetes Is Chronic...1

1.2: Insulin Resistance: The Real Cause Disclosing................... 2

1.3: The Downward Spiral: How the Issue Gets Worse Under Conventional Therapy...3

1.4: A Look Ahead: The Influence of Diet and Intermittent Fasting... 4

CHAPTER 2... 6
An Overview of Insulin and Its Function.............................. 6

2.1: Insulin's Master Switch: How It Controls Blood Sugar.......... 6

2.2: The Body Quits Listening: An Explanation of Insulin Resistance... 7

2.3: The Aftermath - The Significance of Insulin Resistance on Health..8

2.4: Insulin Myths Debunked: Distinguishing Fact from Fiction. 10

CHAPTER 3... 13
The Illusion That Calories Are Inconsequential......................13

3.1: The Calorie Fallacy: Why It Can Be Inaccurate to Focus Only on Calories... 13

3.2: The Carbohydrate Connection: How Insulin Increases Are

    Caused by Carbs.. 14

    3.3: The Benefits of Fat: Why Good Fats Encourage Fullness and Wellness.. 16

    3.4: Putting Protein, Good Fats, and Low-Carb Vegetables First to Create a Balanced Plate.. 17

CHAPTER 4... 20

The Benefits of Sporadic Fasting... 20

    4.1: Learning from Our Ancestors: The Evolutionary Advantages of Fasting.. 20

    4.2: The Cellular Clean-up Team: How Autophagy and Cell Repair Are Encouraged by Fasting... 22

    4.3: Various Fasting Methods: Select the Best One for You...... 23

    4.4: Handling Your Hunger Pangs - Useful Advice to Make Fasting Easier.. 26

CHAPTER 5... 31

Formulating a Customized Course of Care..................................... 31

    5.1: SMART Goal Setting: Identifying Achievement and Monitoring Development.. 31

    5.2: Food Trigger Identification: Understanding Which Foods Cause Blood Sugar Increases.. 33

    5.3: Mastering the Art of Reading Food Labels: A Comprehensive Guide on Carbohydrate and Sugar Content.... 34

    5.4: Creating a Sustainable Way of Life: Choosing Healthful Decisions That Fit Your Schedule... 36

CHAPTER 6... 39

Controlling Body Composition and Weight..................................... 39

6.1: Body Composition's Significance - Why Weight Isn't the Only Consideration.. 39

6.2: Gaining Muscle Mass: How Exercise Increases Fat Burning and Metabolism..41

6.3: The Sleeping Goddess: How Sleep Helps with Hormone Balancing and Weight Control.. 42

6.4: Handling Emotional Eating: Techniques for Handling Tension and Wants..43

CHAPTER 7... 46

Treating Diabetes-Related Complications................................... 46

7.1: Lowering the Risk of Heart Disease: How Diet and Lifestyle Reduce Inflammation and Blood Pressure.............................. 46

7.2: Eye Protection - Preventing Diabetes-Related Vision Loss 48

7.3: Nerve Pain Management: Techniques for Easing Uncomfort and Boosting Life Quality... 49

7.4: Preserving Kidney Function: How Food and Drugs Can Delay Kidney Damage... 51

CHAPTER 8... 54

Managing Diabetes to Lead a Full Life.................................... 54

8.1: Redefining Your Relationship with Food: Savoring Food Fearlessly..54

8.2: Establishing a Network of Support - Locating Motivation and Advocacy... 56

8.3: Embracing Exercise: Selecting Pleasurable and Energizing Activities..57

8.4: Honoring Achievements - Giving Yourself a Praise for

Advancement and Keeping Your Motivation Up..........59

CHAPTER 9..........62

Diabetes Care's Future..........62

9.1: A Change in Perspective: Transitioning to Preventive and Customized Medicine..........62

9.2: Patient Empowerment - Using Information and Knowledge to Take Charge of Your Health..........64

9.3: The Function of Technology - Making Use of Apps and Tools to Aid in Your Travels..........65

9.4: Making a Difference - Creating a Future for Diabetes Treatment and Research..........67

CHAPTER 10..........70

Living Proof: Heartwarming Narratives of Recovery..........70

10.1: Success Stories: Actual People Curing Their Diabetes....70

10.2: Meeting Difficulties Head-On and Solving Problems Along the Way..........72

10.3: Sustainability over the Long Term - Sustaining a Healthful Lifestyle for Life..........74

10.4: A Hope-Filled Story: You Can Reverse Type 2 Diabetes and Govern Your Own Health..........75

ABOUT THE AUTHOR..........76

Disclaimer

This book contains material that is meant to serve as general guidance for managing type 2 diabetes and for educational purposes. It is not meant to serve as a replacement for expert medical advice, diagnosis, or care. When in doubt, always consult your doctor or other certified healthcare expert before making any decisions about a medical problem.

Every effort has been taken by the author and publisher to guarantee the dependability and correctness of the material provided in this book. That being said, recommendations are subject to alter throughout time due to the ongoing evolution of medical knowledge and practices. As a result, the material provided here is not guaranteed to be accurate, full, current, or adequate by the author or publisher.

Dear Amazon and Readers,

Greetings, Readers and Amazon.

In this book, we want to offer important insights and useful guidance on treating type 2 diabetes. Although we are confident in the content's quality and applicability, individual outcomes may differ based on things like health state, following advice, and managing one's own health care. While our goal is to provide readers with inspiration and knowledge, we are unable to control all potential customer reviews or guarantee any particular result. We urge readers to make the most of this book as a tool to deepen their comprehension and have knowledgeable conversations with medical professionals.

We appreciate your consideration of our letter and disclaimer.

Regards,
Harmony Royce

ACKNOWLEDGMENTS

I want to express my sincere gratitude to everyone who helped to write this book on managing and curing diabetes.

We are grateful to the educators, researchers, and healthcare professionals whose knowledge and commitment provide the insightful information presented in these pages. Your dedication to improving diabetes care is incredibly motivating.

I sincerely appreciate everyone who so kindly shared their personal victories over diabetes. For readers everywhere, your bravery and tenacity are an inspiration and a source of hope.

I would especially like to thank my family and friends for their continuous understanding, support, and encouragement along this journey. Your confidence in me and the significance of raising diabetes awareness has been really helpful.

Finally, I would like to thank everyone of the book's

readers for their support and attention. My genuine wish is that the knowledge, suggestions, and anecdotes in these chapters will encourage you to take charge of your own journey toward greater health and wellbeing.

CHAPTER 1

The Big Lie About Type 2 Diabetes

1.1: The Myth - The Reason We Believe Type 2 Diabetes Is Chronic

It has long been believed that type 2 diabetes is a chronic, lifelong illness. A diagnosis can frequently feel like a life sentence because of how deeply embedded this belief is in both the medical community and the general population. There is a widespread misconception that type 2 diabetes is a lifelong condition. The way diabetes is usually treated, the propaganda from pharmaceutical firms, and a general ignorance of the underlying causes of the condition all contribute to this fallacy.

According to conventional understanding, type 2 diabetes is a condition that progressively worsens over time. The fact that patients need higher doses of medicine and may eventually require insulin therapy serves as the basis for this belief. Nevertheless, this viewpoint ignores an important fact: type 2 diabetes's underlying etiology is treatable, if not curable.

1.2: Insulin Resistance: The Real Cause Disclosing

Insulin resistance is a disorder that is at the core of type 2 diabetes. The hormone insulin, which the pancreas produces, enables cells to absorb glucose from the blood and use it as fuel. Elevated blood sugar levels are caused by insulin resistance, a condition in which the body's cells lose their sensitivity to insulin.

Genetics, lifestyle, and nutrition are some of the factors that influence the development of insulin resistance. Fat buildup in the muscles and liver can result from a diet heavy in refined sugars and carbs and a sedentary lifestyle. Insulin resistance develops because of this fat accumulation, which reduces the cells' sensitivity to insulin.

The elevated blood sugar levels associated with type 2 diabetes are primarily caused by insulin resistance. The pancreas produces extra insulin to make up for cells that develop resistance to it. Long-term control over blood sugar levels can be achieved by this compensatory mechanism, but eventually the pancreas may become overworked and less able to generate insulin. Type 2 diabetes is diagnosed as a result of an increase in blood sugar levels.

1.3: The Downward Spiral: How the Issue Gets Worse Under Conventional Therapy

Medication intended to reduce blood sugar levels is a common component of conventional type 2 diabetes treatment. These drugs can effectively treat the symptoms of the condition, but they don't deal with insulin resistance, which is the disease's underlying cause. Certain treatments have the potential to worsen the issue.

For example, people with type 2 diabetes who are on insulin therapy may experience weight gain. This weight gain can exacerbate insulin resistance, especially if it leads to a rise in visceral fat, or fat that is stored around the organs. Patients may thus find themselves in a vicious cycle wherein larger insulin dosages are needed to maintain blood sugar control, but these higher doses further exacerbate insulin resistance.

Furthermore, concentrating only on reducing blood sugar levels may create a false sense of security. A patient's diabetes may seem under control as long as their blood sugar levels are within the desired range. Unfortunately, the condition worsens because this treatment does not address the underlying metabolic abnormality.

1.4: A Look Ahead: The Influence of Diet and Intermittent Fasting

Though conventional therapeutic options present a grim picture, hope is not lost. According to new research, food and intermittent fasting may be crucial for improving type 2 diabetes management and correcting insulin resistance.

By limiting the consumption of foods that raise blood glucose levels, a low-carb diet, for instance, can help lower blood sugar levels. People can lower their body's requirement for insulin to digest glucose and increase their insulin sensitivity by emphasizing whole meals, healthy fats, and sufficient protein.

It has also been demonstrated that intermittent fasting, which alternates between eating and fasting times, might enhance insulin sensitivity and encourage weight loss. The body is compelled to use fat reserves during fasting periods, which can help lower fat deposits in the muscles and liver and increase insulin sensitivity.

Research has demonstrated that a low-carb diet combined with periods of fasting can result in notable improvements in blood sugar regulation and, in certain situations, total remission of type 2 diabetes. Rather than focusing only on treating the symptoms, this strategy targets insulin resistance, the disease's underlying cause.

It is false to assume that type 2 diabetes is an ongoing, incurable illness. Type 2 diabetes can be managed, and even reversed, by recognizing that insulin resistance is the underlying cause of the condition and implementing dietary and intermittent fasting practices. People now have hope and the ability to take charge of their health and well-being because of this paradigm change.

CHAPTER 2

An Overview of Insulin and Its Function

2.1: Insulin's Master Switch: How It Controls Blood Sugar

It's common to refer to insulin as the "master switch" in the body's metabolic operations. This potent hormone, which the pancreatic beta cells produce, is essential for controlling blood sugar levels and ensuring that cells get the energy they require to function.

Upon consumption, the glucose in your meal is converted from the carbs and enters your bloodstream. The pancreas releases insulin in response to an increase in blood glucose levels. Insulin functions as a key, opening cells so that glucose can enter and be used as an energy source. In the absence of insulin, glucose builds up in the blood and can eventually cause high blood sugar levels, which can be dangerous.

Insulin affects protein metabolism and fat storage in addition to helping control blood sugar. Insulin facilitates the conversion of extra glucose into fat for long-term storage and stores it in the liver as glycogen when there is an excess of the sugar. Insulin has several different roles, which emphasize how crucial it is to preserving overall metabolic balance.

2.2: The Body Quits Listening: An Explanation of Insulin Resistance

When the body's cells stop responding to insulin's messages, it can lead to insulin resistance. Consider attempting to open a door with a key that just doesn't fit completely; no matter how hard you try, the door won't open easily. Similar to this, cells that are insulin resistant do not react to insulin as well, which keeps glucose from entering and raises blood sugar levels.

Insulin resistance arises as a result of several circumstances, such as:

1. **Genetics:** Some people are more prone to type 2 diabetes due to a genetic predisposition to insulin resistance.
2. **Diet:** An excessive intake of sweets, processed carbs, and bad fats can cause fat to build up in the muscles and liver, which disrupts insulin signaling.
3. **Sedentary Lifestyle:** Insulin resistance is facilitated by a sedentary lifestyle, which lowers the muscles' capacity to utilize glucose.
4. **Obesity:** Excess body fat, especially visceral fat, causes the release of inflammatory chemicals that disrupt the function of insulin.

Maintaining normal blood sugar levels, the pancreas compensates by generating more insulin as insulin resistance increases. After a while, the pancreas is unable to keep up with this compensatory mechanism, which raises blood sugar levels and causes type 2 diabetes.

2.3: The Aftermath - The Significance of Insulin Resistance on Health

High blood sugar levels are not the only negative health

outcomes that are triggered by insulin resistance. Among them are:

1. **Metabolic Syndrome:** A number of conditions, including high blood pressure, elevated blood sugar, excess abdominal fat, and abnormal cholesterol levels, are associated with metabolic syndrome, one of which is insulin resistance. Type 2 diabetes, heart disease, and stroke are all at increased risk in those with metabolic syndrome.
2. **Cardiovascular Disease:** Atherosclerosis, or the hardening of the arteries, is a result of high insulin levels linked to insulin resistance, which raises the risk of heart attacks and strokes.
3. **Non-Alcoholic Fatty Liver Disease (NAFLD):** Insulin resistance-related excess fat accumulation in the liver can cause inflammation, scarring, and ultimately liver failure.
4. **Polycystic Ovary Syndrome (PCOS):** PCOS is a hormonal condition that affects many women of reproductive age and is characterized by irregular menstrual cycles, excessive hair growth, and infertility. Insulin resistance is connected to PCOS.

5. **Type 2 Diabetes:** When the pancreas is unable to produce enough insulin over time due to persistent insulin resistance, the result is persistently elevated blood sugar levels and the diagnosis of type 2 diabetes.

2.4: Insulin Myths Debunked: Distinguishing Fact from Fiction

Regarding insulin and its function in diabetes, there are a few common myths. Let's discuss and dispel a few of the most widespread myths:

1. **Myth:** People with type 1 diabetes are the only ones who require insulin.
- **Fact:** Many individuals with type 2 diabetes also need insulin to maintain their blood sugar levels when other drugs are not enough, even though insulin therapy is crucial for managing type 1 diabetes.

2. **Myth:** If you take insulin, your diabetes management is a failure.

- **Fact:** Insulin therapy does not indicate a lack of success. It's an essential tool for controlling blood sugar levels and averting issues. The fact that diabetes is a progressing condition is one of many variables influencing the demand for insulin.

3. **Myth:** Insulin is undesirable since it can lead to weight gain and other adverse effects.
- **Truth:** Although insulin use might cause weight gain, this can be controlled with a healthy diet and frequent exercise. The advantages of insulin over any drawbacks are substantial when it comes to regulating blood sugar levels and averting issues.

4. **Myth:** You can never quit taking insulin once you start.
- **Fact:** Some type 2 diabetics can lower or even stop taking insulin by adopting healthier lifestyle practices including eating a balanced diet and getting regular exercise. But you should always perform this under medical supervision.

5. **Myth:** Insulin can be substituted by natural

therapies.
- **Reality:** Although some dietary and lifestyle adjustments can enhance overall health and insulin sensitivity, they cannot take the place of insulin therapy for people who require it. Insulin continues to be a vital component of care for many diabetics.

It is crucial to comprehend the function of insulin and the consequences of insulin resistance in order to manage and possibly even reverse type 2 diabetes. People can take proactive measures toward improved health and well-being by addressing the underlying reasons and dispelling popular beliefs.

CHAPTER 3

The Illusion That Calories Are Inconsequential

3.1: The Calorie Fallacy: Why It Can Be Inaccurate to Focus Only on Calories

Nutritional advice has been dominated for decades by the idea that "calories in, calories out" is the key to managing weight. This oversimplified perspective contends that reaching and maintaining a healthy weight may be accomplished by simply balancing the amount of calories taken and the amount of calories burned through activity. Nevertheless, this viewpoint is deceptive and inadequate.

The notion that all calories are created equal, regardless of their source, is the root of the calorie fallacy. Actually, the body uses calories in a variety of ways depending on what kind they are. For example, the body reacts differently to 100 calories from a sugar-filled soda than it does to 100 calories from a piece of grilled chicken. Sugar-filled beverages have the potential to quickly raise insulin and blood sugar levels, which can result in hunger pangs and fat storage. Conversely, foods high in protein, like chicken, help you feel full and help your muscles heal.

Moreover, the calorie fallacy disregards how different diets affect hormones and metabolism. Important functions for appetite, satiety, and fat storage are played by hormones such as insulin, ghrelin, and leptin. Regardless of calorie content, diets high in refined carbs can interfere with these hormonal signals, causing overeating and weight gain.

3.2: The Carbohydrate Connection: How Insulin Increases Are Caused by Carbs

Specifically, processed and refined carbohydrates have a major effect on insulin and blood sugar levels. Upon ingestion, carbohydrates are converted to glucose and absorbed into the bloodstream. The hormone insulin, which aids cells in absorbing glucose for use as fuel or storage, is released by the pancreas in response to this.

But not every carbohydrate is made equally. Simple carbs, like those in white bread and sugary snacks, are easily absorbed and digested, which results in sharp increases in insulin and blood sugar levels. A cycle of energy highs and lows, heightened appetite, and fat storage, especially around the abdomen, can result from these increases.

Whole grains, veggies, and legumes are good sources of complex carbs, which raise insulin and blood sugar levels more gradually. They provide a consistent energy source and aid in preserving stable blood sugar levels since they are more slowly absorbed and digested. In addition to encouraging sensations of fullness, this delayed digestion lowers the chance of overindulging.

Another important aspect of the carbohydrate relationship is the function of insulin in fat storage. The body is more likely to retain extra glucose as fat when insulin levels are high, especially in the liver and abdomen. Over time, this can exacerbate the issue and raise the risk of type 2 diabetes and metabolic syndrome by causing cells to become less sensitive to insulin's signals, a condition known as insulin resistance.

3.3: The Benefits of Fat: Why Good Fats Encourage Fullness and Wellness

Dietary fat was demonized for a long time as the main cause of heart disease and weight gain. Nonetheless, current studies have demonstrated that good fats are critical for satiety and wellbeing in addition to being vital for general health.

Many body processes depend on healthy fats, which can be found in nuts, seeds, avocados, and olive oil. They serve as an enduring source of energy, are essential parts of cell membranes, and aid in the absorption of fat-soluble vitamins (A, D, E, and K). In contrast to carbs, which can lead to abrupt increases and decreases in blood sugar levels, fats offer a consistent, prolonged release of energy.

Healthy fats' capacity to increase satiety is among its most important advantages. Because fats break down more slowly than carbohydrates, they contribute to your feeling full and content in between meals. This can stop overeating and lower total calorie intake.

Furthermore, studies have demonstrated the anti-inflammatory qualities of good fats, which may help lower the chance of developing chronic illnesses like arthritis and heart disease. They also contribute to maintaining the health of the brain; omega-3 fatty acids, in particular, are essential for mental and cognitive function.

3.4: Putting Protein, Good Fats, and Low-Carb Vegetables First to Create a Balanced Plate

A sensible strategy to enhance metabolic health and sustain a healthy weight is to arrange your food in a balanced plate with an emphasis on protein, healthy fats, and low-carb veggies. How to make such a plate is as follows:

1. **Make Protein Your Top Priority:** Protein is necessary for immune system support, tissue growth and repair, and muscle mass maintenance. Additionally, it encourages satiety, which aids in reducing overall calorie consumption and controlling appetite. Every meal should have some form of lean protein, such as beans, tofu, fish, poultry, or eggs.

2. **Incorporate Healthy Fats:** As previously indicated, healthy fats encourage satiety and long-lasting energy. Incorporate foods like avocados, almonds, seeds, olive oil, and fatty seafood like salmon into your diet as sources of healthful fats. You can cook these fats with veggies, add them to salads, or eat them as snacks.

3. **Fill Up on Low-Carb Vegetables:** Vegetables are low in calories and high in fiber, antioxidants, and other nutrients. They also barely affect blood sugar levels. Give special attention to non-starchy veggies such as zucchini, peppers, cauliflower, broccoli, and leafy greens. You can eat these veggies fresh in salads or steam, roast, or cook them.

4. **Minimize Processed and Refined Carbohydrates:** Cut back on processed and refined carbs such white bread, spaghetti, pastries, and sugary snacks. These foods have the potential to quickly raise insulin and blood sugar levels, which can increase appetite and promote fat accumulation.

5. **Remain Hydrated:** A balanced diet must include adequate hydration. Water promotes overall health, nutrient absorption, and digestion. Drink lots of water throughout the day, and avoid overindulging in sugary or caffeinated beverages.

You may support your body's metabolic processes, enhance insulin sensitivity, and reach a healthier weight without constantly monitoring your caloric intake by emphasizing nutrient-dense foods and maintaining macronutrient balance. This strategy prioritizes long-term health and wellbeing by emphasizing dietary quality over quantity.

CHAPTER 4

The Benefits of Sporadic Fasting

4.1: Learning from Our Ancestors: The Evolutionary Advantages of Fasting

The idea of intermittent fasting is not new. As a matter of fact, it has its roots in our evolutionary past. Unlike us, our predecessors did not always have access to food; they went through times of plenty and famine. Our bodies become accustomed to going for extended periods of time without food thanks to this eating and fasting routine that formed our metabolism.

Our ancestors' bodies adapted to use stored energy effectively during periods of food scarcity. They would consume food when it was available and store the extra energy as fat. Their bodies would use these fat stores as fuel when they were fasting. They were able to live and prosper in circumstances where food availability was unpredictable because of their cycle of eating and fasting.

These days, intermittent fasting imitates this ancestral feeding schedule and has multiple evolutionary advantages:

1. **Metabolic Flexibility:** Fasting improves metabolic flexibility by teaching the body to alternate between burning fat and glucose for energy. This capacity to use various energy sources effectively contributes to the preservation of energy balance and the avoidance of metabolic disorders.

2. **Insulin Sensitivity:** By lowering the frequency of insulin spikes, intermittent fasting enhances insulin sensitivity. The body's cells react to insulin more effectively when there are fewer insulin spikes, which reduces the likelihood of insulin resistance and type 2 diabetes.

3. **Hormonal Balance:** Growth hormone, which encourages fat burning and muscle preservation, and norepinephrine, which raises metabolic rate and calorie expenditure, are among the hormones that

fasting favorably influences.

4.2: The Cellular Clean-up Team: How Autophagy and Cell Repair Are Encouraged by Fasting

The capacity of intermittent fasting to promote autophagy—a mechanism by which the body's cells recycle damaged components for energy—is among its most persuasive advantages. Greek word autophagy means "self-eating," and it is an essential process for cellular upkeep and repair.

During a fast, the body perceives limited energy supply and triggers autophagy. This procedure aids in:

1. **Remove Cellular Debris:** Autophagy eliminates faulty or damaged cell parts, avoiding the build-up of waste that can exacerbate illness and aging.

2. **Recycle Nutrients**: Autophagy recycles vital nutrients by disassembling damaged components, giving the body the building blocks it needs for cellular regeneration and repair.

3. **Improve Immune Function:** By eliminating pathogens and damaged cells, autophagy helps the immune system function better and helps the body fight off infections and illnesses.

4. **Protect Against Neurodegeneration:** Misfolded proteins and damaged mitochondria, which can exacerbate neurodegenerative illnesses like Alzheimer's and Parkinson's, can be eliminated by autophagy.

5. **Intermittent fasting** improves overall health and longevity by lowering the risk of chronic diseases and strengthening the body's ability to withstand stress through the promotion of autophagy and cellular repair.

4.3: Various Fasting Methods: Select the Best One for You

There are various approaches to intermittent fasting, and each has advantages and disadvantages of its own. Finding a technique that works for your lifestyle and health objectives is crucial. Here are a few well-liked methods for intermittent fasting:

1. **16/8 Method:** This plan calls for eating all of your meals within an 8-hour window and fasting for 16 hours. For instance, you may fast from 8 p.m. to noon the following day and eat between noon and 8pm Due to its ability to accommodate a daily feeding window that works with most schedules, this is one of the most widely used and sustained forms of fasting.

2. **5:2 Diet:** This plan calls for eating regularly five days a week and drastically cutting calories (around 500–600) on two non-consecutive days. For individuals who would rather have fewer fasting days, this approach may work, although it does necessitate careful preparation to guarantee sufficient nutrition on fasting days.

3. **Eat-Stop-Eat:** This tactic calls for one or two 24-hour fasts per week. For instance, you may stop

eating at 7 p.m. and start eating again at 7 p.m. the following day. Even though it works well, this approach can be difficult for newcomers and may need some incremental adjustment.

4. **Alternate-Day Fasting:** This method switches up the days you eat and fast. You either follow a strict fast (approximately 500 calories) or eat very little on fasting days. Although it could be challenging to follow this strategy consistently over time, it can be useful for promoting metabolic health and losing weight.

5. **Warrior Diet:** This plan consists of consuming a single, substantial meal within a 4-hour eating window at night and little portions of fresh fruits and vegetables during the day. It may be appropriate for people who would rather only eat one large meal a day and is based on the eating habits of ancient warriors.

6. **Spontaneous Meal Skipping:** You can skip meals whenever it's convenient for you, as opposed to

adhering to a set fasting schedule. For people who are unfamiliar with intermittent fasting, this method can be an excellent place to start because it offers flexibility and the benefits of fasting.

Think on your lifestyle, work schedule, and personal preferences while selecting a fasting plan. Paying attention to your body and making necessary adjustments is crucial. Some people might think that some approaches are more practical or efficient than others. Whichever method is used, intermittent fasting has several health advantages, including better metabolic health, cellular regeneration, and weight management.

4.4: Handling Your Hunger Pangs - Useful Advice to Make Fasting Easier

At first, intermittent fasting may be difficult, particularly when adjusting to times when you don't eat. The following useful advice can help you get past hunger sensations and make fasting more tolerable:

1. **Remain Hydrated:** During fasting times, drinking

black coffee, herbal teas, or water will help you stay hydrated and reduce hunger. Hydration is important since sometimes thirst is confused with hunger.

2. **Start Slowly:** If you've never fasted before, think about extending your fasting window gradually. As your body adjusts, progressively increase the fasting duration from a lesser starting point—12 hours, for example.

3. **Stay Busy :** Take part in activities that divert your attention from food-related concerns. This can involve employment, interests, physical activity, or hanging out with pals.

4. **Acquire Electrolytes:** During fasting, low-calorie electrolyte beverages or supplements can assist preserve electrolyte balance and reduce sensations of exhaustion or weakness.

5. **Include Fiber-Rich meals:** Give fiber-rich meals like fruits, vegetables, and whole grains top priority during your eating window. Fiber makes fasting

periods more comfortable by promoting satiety and assisting in blood sugar regulation.

6. **Listen to Your Body:** Pay heed to the cues that your body gives you. You can change your fasting schedule or break your fast early with a light, nourishing meal if you feel extremely hungry or ill while fasting.

7. **Select Nutrient-Dense Foods:** During your eating window, choose meals that are high in vitamins, minerals, and antioxidants. Foods high in nutrients can assist maintain energy levels and lessen cravings when fasting.

8. **Practice Mindfulness:** To reduce stress and enhance your connection with hunger cues, incorporate mindfulness practices like yoga, meditation, or deep breathing.

9. **Acquire Enough Sleep:** Enough sleep promotes general health and controls appetite hormones. Aim for 7 to 9 hours of good sleep every night to get the

most out of fasting.

10. **Be Patient:** Give your body some time to become used to sporadic fasting. Hunger sensations may not go away for a few weeks while your body adjusts to the new food schedule.

You can facilitate the shift to intermittent fasting and increase its efficacy as a strategy for enhancing metabolic health and general well-being by putting these helpful suggestions into practice. Keep in mind that not everyone can follow an intermittent fasting program, so before making any big dietary or fasting adjustments, speak with a healthcare provider.

By drawing on our evolutionary past, intermittent fasting is a potent tool that supports hormonal balance, insulin sensitivity, and metabolic flexibility. Fasting promotes cellular repair and autophagy, which enhance general health and longevity. With so many different fasting techniques available, it's critical to select one that best suits your objectives and way of life. Adopting intermittent fasting can result in notable enhancements to one's health, overall wellbeing, and standard of living.

CHAPTER 5

Formulating a Customized Course of Care

Making a customized treatment plan is essential to successfully managing your health, particularly if you have type 2 diabetes or other related illnesses. You will be guided through the necessary procedures in this chapter to customize a strategy that meets your lifestyle and health objectives.

5.1: SMART Goal Setting: Identifying Achievement and Monitoring Development

The first stage in developing an effective treatment plan is to set SMART goals, or Specific, Measurable, Achievable, Relevant, and Time-bound:

1. **Specific:** Establish precise, well-defined objectives pertaining to your well-being, such reaching a desired weight, enhancing blood sugar control, or

stepping up your physical activity.

2. **Measurable:** Create standards to monitor development. This could include keeping an eye on blood sugar levels every day, documenting weight loss, or keeping track of exercise minutes.

3. **Achievable:** Make sure your goals are doable and reasonable. Segment more ambitious objectives into more doable, smaller steps to keep momentum and enthusiasm high.

4. **Relevant:** Make sure your objectives complement your lifestyle and overall health goals. Think about how reaching these objectives will improve your health in the long run.

5. **Time-bound:** Assign deadlines to each target. This establishes a sense of urgency and offers a precise benchmark for assessment and modification.

You give yourself the power to take proactive measures toward efficiently managing your condition and tracking your progress by setting SMART goals.

5.2: Food Trigger Identification: Understanding Which Foods Cause Blood Sugar Increases

It's critical to comprehend how various foods impact your blood sugar levels if you have type 2 diabetes. Determine and keep an eye out for meal triggers that may result in blood glucose spikes:

1. **Carbohydrate Impact:** The biggest influence on blood sugar levels comes from carbohydrates. distinct carbs have distinct effects on blood sugar, such as simple sugars versus complex sugars.

2. **Glycemic Index (GI):** Whole foods with a low GI release glucose more gradually, those with a high GI produce sharp rises in blood sugar levels. Make an effort to eat a lot of low-GI foods, such as legumes, whole grains, and non-starchy veggies.

3. **Individual Response:** Observe the reactions that various foods have on your body. To keep track of

how different meals impact your blood sugar levels, keep a food journal or use a glucose monitor.

4. **Portion Control:** Consuming a lot of healthful food can have an impact on blood sugar levels. To keep blood sugar levels steady, spread out your carbohydrate intake throughout the day and practice portion management.

Being aware of your food triggers will enable you to make well-informed dietary decisions that promote stable blood sugar regulation and general health.

5.3: Mastering the Art of Reading Food Labels: A Comprehensive Guide on Carbohydrate and Sugar Content

Learn how to properly read food labels so that you may control your consumption of carbohydrates and make wise decisions:

1. **Total Carbohydrates:** Take note of how many carbohydrates there are in each dish. This contains

carbs that affect blood sugar levels, fiber, and sugars.

2. **Fiber Content:** Choose foods that are high in dietary fiber because it increases satiety and inhibits the absorption of glucose. Try to get as least 25–30 grams of fiber from whole foods each day.

3. **Sugar Content:** Determine whether processed goods have additional sugars. Select foods that have the fewest added sugars and concentrate on naturally sweet foods like fruits.

4. **Servings per Container:** To prevent overindulging and precisely determine your daily intake of carbohydrates, make sure you are aware of the serving size and quantity per container.

5. **Ingredients List:** Look for artificial additives and hidden sugars in the ingredients list. Whenever possible, select dishes made from simple, natural foods.

You can make decisions that support optimal blood sugar

management and are in line with your dietary goals by reading food labels.

5.4: Creating a Sustainable Way of Life: Choosing Healthful Decisions That Fit Your Schedule

A sustainable way of living is essential for long-term health and wellbeing. Think about the following methods for incorporating healthful practices into your everyday schedule:

1. **Regular Physical Activity:** Include regular exercise in your weekly routine, such as weight training, swimming, or walking. Try to get in at least 150 minutes a week of moderate-to-intense activity, or as advised by your physician.

2. **Meal Planning and Preparation:** To prevent impulsive eating decisions, plan balanced meals and snacks in advance. Meal preparation and batch cooking can ensure that wholesome meals are always available while also saving time.

3. **Stress Management:** Engage in relaxing activities, yoga, meditation, deep breathing, or other stress-relieving practices. Both blood sugar levels and general health can be impacted by prolonged stress.

4. **Quality Sleep:** Make maintaining proper sleep hygiene a top priority to promote both general health and healthy metabolic function. Aim for seven to nine hours of good sleep every night.

5. **Social Support:** Be in the company of encouraging friends, relatives, or neighborhood associations. Talking to people about your objectives and difficulties might help you stay motivated and accountable.

6. **Regular Monitoring and Check-ins:** Make an appointment for routine check-ins with your medical team to discuss any concerns or inquiries, monitor treatment plans, and assess progress.

Making small adjustments that you can stick with over

time is the key to creating a sustainable lifestyle. You may effectively control type 2 diabetes and enhance your overall quality of life by making healthy decisions on a regular basis.

Developing a sustainable lifestyle, recognizing dietary triggers, reading food labels, and creating SMART goals are all important components of developing a customized treatment plan for type 2 diabetes. You may maximize your health, accomplish your goals, and have a full life while efficiently managing your condition by being proactive and making educated decisions. Speak with your healthcare professional to create a plan that suits your particular requirements and promotes long-term health.

CHAPTER 6

Controlling Body Composition and Weight

For general well-being and the management of illnesses like type 2 diabetes, reaching and maintaining a healthy weight is essential. In order to promote optimal health, this chapter examines a number of weight management topics with a particular emphasis on body composition, muscle mass, sleep, and emotional eating techniques.

6.1: Body Composition's Significance - Why Weight Isn't the Only Consideration

The percentage of fat mass and lean mass (bone, muscle, and water) in the body is referred to as body composition. For a number of reasons, body composition should be taken into account instead of merely body weight.

1. **Health Risks:** Being overweight raises the chance of developing chronic illnesses such type 2 diabetes, heart disease, and stroke, particularly visceral fat

surrounding organs.

2. **Metabolic Health:** Insulin sensitivity, hormonal balance, and metabolic rate are all impacted by body composition. Maintaining metabolic health and burning calories depend heavily on lean muscle mass.

3. **Fitness and Functionality:** The strength, range of motion, and general physical performance are all supported by muscle mass. Sustaining your muscular mass is crucial to preserving your freedom and standard of living as you get older.

4. **Body Image and Confidence:** Regardless of the number on the scale, focusing on body composition rather than just weight will help foster a positive body image and increase self-esteem.

A weight-management strategy that emphasizes decreasing fat mass while maintaining or increasing lean muscle mass can be more effectively tailored with the understanding and monitoring of body composition.

6.2: Gaining Muscle Mass: How Exercise Increases Fat Burning and Metabolism

To increase metabolism, support fat loss, and build and maintain muscle mass, exercise—especially resistance training—is essential.

1. **Metabolic Boost**: Compared to fat tissue, muscle tissue burns more calories at rest due to its higher metabolic activity. Strength training increases muscular mass, which improves metabolism and aids in maintaining a healthy weight.

2. **Fat Burning**: Exercise increases insulin sensitivity and encourages the oxidation of fat, particularly high-intensity interval training (HIIT) and resistance training. This can help improve overall body composition and reduce visceral fat.

3. **Strength and Functionality**: Increasing muscle strength enhances functional skills like lifting, carrying, and balancing, all of which are necessary

for day-to-day tasks and injury prevention.

4. **Bone Health:** Resistance exercise is especially important as you age because it maintains bone density and lowers the chance of osteoporosis.

To optimize health advantages and encourage muscle growth, combine resistance training, cardiovascular activity, and flexibility training into your program.

6.3: The Sleeping Goddess: How Sleep Helps with Hormone Balancing and Weight Control

Good sleep is crucial for general health and has a big impact on hormone balance and weight control:

1. **Hormonal Regulation:** Sleep affects the hormones leptin and ghrelin, which regulate hunger and satiety. These hormones are disturbed by insufficient sleep, which increases hunger and creates desires for high-calorie foods.

2. **Metabolic Function:** Inadequate sleep can affect

insulin sensitivity and glucose metabolism, which can lead to weight gain and insulin resistance.

3. **Recovery and Repair:** Sleep has a critical role in the growth, healing, and repair of muscles. It enhances physical performance and lowers the chance of injury when working out.

4. **Stress Reduction:** Getting enough sleep lowers stress levels and enhances emotional health, which can help people make smart food choices and avoid emotional eating.

To ensure restful sleep and support general health, establish a consistent sleep schedule, develop a calming nighttime routine, and improve your sleeping environment.

6.4: Handling Emotional Eating: Techniques for Handling Tension and Wants

Stress, boredom, or other emotions can lead to emotional eating, which can undermine attempts to control weight instead of satiating hunger. Among the techniques to control emotional eating are:

1. **Identify Triggers:** Be aware of the emotional factors, such as stress, boredom, or social circumstances, that lead to eating. To monitor your eating habits and feelings, keep a food journal.

2. **Find Alternatives:** Create better coping strategies for stress, like physical activity, mindfulness, engaging in a hobby, or speaking with a friend. Activities that satisfy your emotions without involving food can take the place of emotional eating.

3. **Mindful Eating:** Slow down, enjoy every bite, and pay attention to your body's hunger signals. This encourages appreciation of meals and helps prevent overeating.

4. **Healthy Food Choices:** Fill your kitchen with filling, nutrient-dense foods that help you achieve your health objectives. Snack on foods high in fiber, protein, and good fats to help control blood sugar

and reduce cravings.

5. **Seek Support:** To examine emotional triggers and create more healthy coping mechanisms for stress and emotions, get in touch with a therapist, counselor, or support group.

You may effectively improve your health outcomes and accomplish sustainable weight control by addressing emotional eating and using techniques that enhance muscle mass, sleep quality, and overall body composition.

For general health and well-being, controlling weight and body composition is crucial, particularly for those with diseases like type 2 diabetes. You may maximize your health and reach long-term weight management objectives by addressing emotional eating, managing body composition, prioritizing quality sleep, increasing muscle mass through exercise, and addressing body image. Speak with medical experts to create a customized plan that fits your requirements and encourages a healthy way of living.

CHAPTER 7

Treating Diabetes-Related Complications

Diabetes can result in a number of problems that impact different body areas. This chapter focuses on methods for managing or reversing these issues through dietary adjustments, medical procedures, and lifestyle modifications.

7.1: Lowering the Risk of Heart Disease: How Diet and Lifestyle Reduce Inflammation and Blood Pressure

Diabetes patients are at a high risk of developing heart disease. This risk can be considerably decreased by controlling blood pressure and inflammation through dietary and lifestyle modifications:

1. **Healthy Diet:** Make a heart-healthy diet high in whole grains, fruits, vegetables, lean meats, and healthy fats (such as fish's omega-3 fatty acids). To strengthen your heart, cut back on sodium,

cholesterol, trans fats, and saturated fats.

2. **Regular Exercise:** Exercise on a regular basis to keep your weight in check, enhance circulation, and lower blood pressure. Try to get in at least 150 minutes a week of strength training in addition to moderate-intensity cardiovascular exercise.

3. **Blood Glucose Control:** To lessen inflammation and damage to blood vessels and organs, maintain ideal blood glucose levels. Keep a frequent eye on your blood sugar levels and follow your treatment plan.

4. **Stop Smoking:** Heart disease risk is increased by smoking. Giving up smoking can enhance general health and heart health.

5. **Medication Management:** To effectively manage blood pressure, cholesterol, and blood glucose levels, adhere to your healthcare provider's recommendations regarding medications.

You can reduce your risk of heart disease and enhance your cardiovascular health by putting these methods into practice, which is essential for managing the problems of diabetes.

7.2: Eye Protection - Preventing Diabetes-Related Vision Loss

Diabetic retinopathy and other visual problems are associated with diabetes. Use these precautions to keep your vision safe:

1. **Regular Eye Exams:** To identify early indicators of diabetic eye problems, make an appointment for routine, thorough eye exams with an eye specialist.

2. **Blood Sugar Control:** To guard against harm to the blood vessels in the retina, keep your blood sugar levels steady. It is imperative to monitor and maintain blood glucose levels consistently.

3. **Blood Pressure Management:** Lower high blood pressure because it can exacerbate other eye

disorders, such as diabetic retinopathy.

4. **Stop Smoking**: Diabetes eye disease is more likely to develop in smokers. Giving up smoking can help you keep your eyes and general health safe.

5. **Eye Protection:** To shield your eyes from sunlight, injuries, and irritants, wear safety goggles and sunglasses with UV protection as needed.

To protect eyesight and avoid consequences from diabetic eye disease, early detection and proactive management are essential.

7.3: Nerve Pain Management: Techniques for Easing Uncomfort and Boosting Life Quality

Diabetic neuropathy may result in discomfort and agony in the nerves. Use these tactics to treat nerve pain:

1. **Blood Sugar Control:** Nerve injury can be avoided or postponed with stable blood glucose levels. Keep an eye on your blood sugar levels and adhere to your

treatment plan.

2. **Medication Management:** Your physician may recommend antidepressants, anticonvulsants, or analgesics to treat your pain. Observe the advice of your healthcare practitioner and report any adverse effects.

3. **Foot Care:** Because diabetic neuropathy can cause decreased sensation, check your feet every day for cuts, blisters, or sores. To avoid issues, proper foot care and routine podiatry visits are crucial.

4. **Physical Therapy:** Perform physical therapy exercises to enhance muscle balance, strength, and flexibility. These improvements can reduce discomfort in the nerves and increase range of motion.

5. **Alternative Therapies**: To reduce nerve pain and enhance quality of life, think about complementary therapies like acupuncture, massage therapy, or biofeedback.

To effectively manage nerve pain, a multidisciplinary strategy that is customized to your specific needs and symptoms must be used.

7.4: Preserving Kidney Function: How Food and Drugs Can Delay Kidney Damage

Diabetic nephropathy, or kidney disease, is mostly caused by diabetes. Use these tactics to safeguard kidney health:

1. **Blood Sugar Control:** Manage blood sugar levels to shield the vulnerable blood vessels in the kidneys from harm. Keep a careful eye on your blood sugar levels and adhere to your treatment plan.

2. **Blood Pressure Management:** Control elevated blood pressure to lessen the kidneys' burden. Medication may be prescribed by your healthcare professional in order to successfully control blood pressure.

3. **Kidney-favorable Diet:** Follow a diet low in

phosphorus, potassium, and sodium that is favorable to the kidneys. As directed by your healthcare professional, cut back on protein to lessen the strain on your kidneys.

4. **Regular Monitoring:** Use blood and urine testing to regularly check kidney function. Timely intervention and management of renal illness are made possible by early identification.

5. **Stop Smoking:** For people with diabetes, smoking causes kidney damage more quickly. Giving up smoking can enhance general health and delay the course of renal disease.

You can effectively manage renal issues connected to diabetes and preserve kidney function by implementing these techniques into your daily routine and collaborating closely with your healthcare team.

Diabetes problems must be managed and reversed using a proactive strategy that includes dietary changes, ongoing observation, and medication therapies. Diabetes can improve quality of life and lessen its effects on general health by concentrating on heart disease risk reduction, eye protection, nerve pain management, and kidney health maintenance. To create a customized plan that meets your unique demands and promotes long-term well-being, confer with medical experts.

CHAPTER 8

Managing Diabetes to Lead a Full Life

Diabetes does not have to prevent you from leading a full and active life. In order to improve general well-being, we discuss ways to enjoy living with diabetes, with an emphasis on nutrition, social networks, physical activity, and acknowledging accomplishments.

8.1: Redefining Your Relationship with Food: Savoring Food Fearlessly

Maintaining your health and enjoying meals while treating diabetes requires redefining your relationship with food:

1. **Balance and Variety:** Adopt a diet full of entire grains, fruits, vegetables, lean meats, healthy fats, and balanced nutrients. Eat a range of foods to guarantee nutrient intake and avoid boredom.

2. **Mindful Eating:** Engage in mindful eating by focusing on signs of hunger, appreciating every bite, and putting distractions out of your mind. This promotes a healthier relationship with food and helps avoid overindulging.

3. **Carbohydrate Management**: Keep an eye on your intake of carbs and go for complex carbohydrates like whole grains and legumes, which release glucose gradually. Distribute your daily intake of carbohydrates and take into account portion sizes.

4. **Adaptability and Moderation:** Give your diet some adaptability while maintaining moderation. Periodic treats are OK as long as they are balanced with nutritious foods and appropriate insulin administration.

5. **Education and Planning**: Learn about diabetic meal planning and nutrition. Create a customized meal plan that suits your preferences and lifestyle by working with a certified dietitian or other healthcare professional.

You can eat with confidence and efficiently manage your diabetes if you approach food with understanding, mindfulness, and balance.

8.2: Establishing a Network of Support - Locating Motivation and Advocacy

Creating a solid support network is essential for managing diabetes and mental health:

1. **Family and Friends:** Talk about your journey with loving family and friends who can offer support, empathy, and useful advice.

2. **Support Groups:** To meet people going through similar struggles, sign up for an online or in-person diabetes support group. These support groups provide compassion, common experiences, and insightful advice on managing diabetes.

3. **Healthcare Team:** Develop a cooperative connection with the physicians, nurses, dietitians,

and diabetes educators that make up your healthcare team. They are able to offer direction, instruction, and customized treatment programs.

4. **Educational Programs:** To improve your understanding, abilities, and self-assurance in managing diabetes, participate in diabetes education programs and workshops. These programs frequently provide peer support, tools, and resources.

5. **Advocacy:** Take up the cause of other diabetics as well as yourself. Promote the availability of high-quality healthcare, surroundings that are conducive to diabetes management, and tools that enhance diabetes knowledge and care.

Your capacity to thrive with diabetes is enhanced when you have a supporting network that offers possibilities for advocacy, practical counsel, and emotional strength.

8.3: Embracing Exercise: Selecting Pleasurable and Energizing Activities

Maintaining cardiovascular health, controlling diabetes, and boosting general wellbeing all depend on regular exercise:

1. **Select Pleasurable Activities:** Whether it's dancing, swimming, cycling, walking, or team sports, choose physical activities that you look forward to and enjoy. Exercise remains interesting and long-lasting with variety.

2. **Set Realistic Goals:** Set attainable exercise objectives, including stepping up daily, getting more flexible, or finishing a fitness challenge. To stay inspired, monitor your development and acknowledge your accomplishments.

3. **Incorporate Strength Training:** To strengthen muscles, enhance metabolism, and promote bone health, incorporate resistance training activities. Aim for two or more sessions a week that concentrate on your main muscle groups.

4. **Mind-Body Exercises:** To lower stress, increase

flexibility, and improve general well being, include mind-body exercises like yoga, tai chi, or Pilates. These activities encourage calmness of mind and relaxation.

5. **Consistency and Routine:** Create a consistent workout regimen that works with your tastes and timetable. To get the long-term advantages of physical activity for managing diabetes, consistency is essential.

Frequent exercise not only lowers blood sugar but also improves mood, eases stress, and increases general vigor.

8.4: Honoring Achievements - Giving Yourself a Praise for Advancement and Keeping Your Motivation Up

Recognizing accomplishments, no matter how modest, inspires persistence and strengthens beneficial diabetes management practices:

1. **Acknowledge accomplishments:** Highlight and celebrate successes like achieving blood sugar

targets, keeping a healthy weight, or forming new lifestyle practices.

2. **Non-Food Rewards:** Treat yourself to non-food indulgences that support your health objectives, such as a day at the spa, new exercise equipment, or a purchase for a hobby.

3. **Track Progress:** Record your accomplishments and significant anniversaries in a journal or online tracker. Think back on your progress and the constructive adjustments you've made.

4. **Share Achievements:** Convey your accomplishments to the diabetes community, your medical team, and your support network. Sharing a celebration with others motivates them and strengthens your bond.

5. **Remain Motivated:** Make the most of holidays to rekindle your enthusiasm and make fresh resolutions for ongoing advancements in diabetes care and general well-being.

You may develop a positive outlook and resilience in controlling your diabetes and live a full and active life by acknowledging your accomplishments and staying motivated.

Having a lively life with diabetes means embracing food fearlessly, establishing a solid support network, getting regular exercise, and acknowledging and appreciating small victories along the way. You may improve your overall health, maintain your best possible well-being, and manage your diabetes well by adopting these tactics into your daily routine and taking a holistic approach to diabetes care. To ensure a satisfying life with diabetes, work with your healthcare team to customize these techniques to meet your specific requirements and objectives.

CHAPTER 9

Diabetes Care's Future

The field of diabetes care is changing quickly, with opportunities for breakthroughs in patient empowerment, prevention, individualized treatment, technological integration, and advocacy. We examine how diabetes care will develop in the future, emphasizing how patient empowerment, technology developments, paradigm shifts, and advocacy initiatives will influence the industry.

9.1: A Change in Perspective: Transitioning to Preventive and Customized Medicine

A paradigm shift towards proactive, individualized treatments that focus early intervention and prevention characterizes the future of diabetes care:

1. **Preventative Medicine:** The focus is on preventing diabetes by altering lifestyle choices, screening at an

early age, and implementing interventions that address risk factors such as genetic predisposition, obesity, and sedentary lifestyle.

2. **Personalized Treatment Plans:** Thanks to developments in genomics and biomarker research, patients can now receive customized care that takes into account their unique genetic makeup, lifestyle choices, and rate of illness progression.

3. **Predictive Analytics:** Predictive analytics and artificial intelligence (AI) are used to identify high-risk patients, forecast the course of a disease, and optimize treatment plans before complications occur.

4. **Integrated Healthcare Models:** Coordinating efforts amongst endocrinologists, nutritionists, psychologists, and primary care physicians to provide complete, coordinated care that takes into account both the psychological and physical elements of managing diabetes.

Healthcare systems can move toward proactive treatment that enhances patient outcomes and lowers healthcare costs related to diabetic complications by adopting preventative strategies and tailored therapy.

9.2: Patient Empowerment - Using Information and Knowledge to Take Charge of Your Health

Providing patients with information and tools is essential for managing their diabetes effectively and leading a better quality of life:

1. **Patient Education:** Extensive diabetes education programs that offer current knowledge on medication administration, physical exercise, diet, and self-care methods.

2. **Shared Decision Making:** Promoting collaborative decision-making between patients and medical professionals while taking into account each patient's unique preferences, values, and treatment objectives.

3. **Health Literacy:** Advancing health literacy via

easily comprehensible and easily accessible resources, such as online forums, workshops, and support groups.

4. **Self-Monitoring Tools:** Monitoring blood glucose levels, medication adherence, food, and exercise with self-monitoring gadgets like continuous glucose monitors (CGMs) and smartphone apps.

Healthcare professionals can promote a collaborative environment that improves treatment adherence, self-management abilities, and general well-being by giving patients the freedom to actively participate in their care.

9.3: The Function of Technology - Making Use of Apps and Tools to Aid in Your Travels

Technology is essential to the transformation of diabetes care because it provides patients with cutting-edge tools and applications to help them along the way:

1. **Continuous Glucose Monitoring (CGM):** CGMs

lower the risk of hypo- and hyperglycemia by providing real-time glucose measurements, trends, and warnings. This allows for proactive control.

2. **Insulin Delivery Systems:** To improve accuracy and convenience, automated insulin delivery systems (closed-loop systems) and sophisticated insulin pumps modify insulin dosage in response to CGM data.

3. **Telemedicine:** Increasing access to specialized treatment and lowering obstacles to healthcare through the development of telemedicine systems for remote consultations, monitoring, and education.

4. **Mobile Applications:** Patients can effectively manage their diabetes and practice self-care by using mobile apps for meal planning, activity tracking, medication reminders, and virtual support groups.

5. **Artificial Intelligence (AI):** AI algorithms are integrated for early detection of issues connected to diabetes, predictive analytics, and individualized

therapy recommendations.

Healthcare professionals can improve patient involvement, optimize diabetes treatment, and foster ongoing improvement in care delivery and outcomes by utilizing technology.

9.4: Making a Difference - Creating a Future for Diabetes Treatment and Research

In order to support research projects, influence legislation, and increase access to cutting-edge diabetes care tools and treatments, advocacy is crucial.

1. **Public Awareness Campaigns:** Use media attention, community outreach, and public campaigns to spread the word about diabetes prevention, management, and the value of early intervention.

2. **Policy Advocacy:** Make the case for laws that promote diabetes prevention initiatives, reasonable drug availability, and payment for diabetes-related

goods and services.

3. **Research Funding:** Provide financial support for studies on diabetes, clinical trials, and novel treatments meant to enhance patient outcomes and discover a cure.

4. **Patient Advocacy Groups:** Work together with patient advocacy groups to promote patient-centered care models, address healthcare disparities, and elevate the voices of patients.

5. **Global Health Initiatives:** Work together to address diabetes as a public health priority, especially in low-income and underserved populations.

Stakeholders may promote scientific advancements, impact healthcare policies, and enhance outcomes for people with diabetes globally by pushing for change.

Transformational advances toward preventative and individualized medication, patient empowerment via technology and information, and advocacy for research improvements and legislative changes are what will define diabetes care in the future. Healthcare systems can improve patient outcomes, improve diabetes treatment, and eventually work toward a world where diabetes is effectively avoided, managed, and one day eradicated by embracing these developments and teamwork. Take part in advocacy campaigns, interact with healthcare practitioners, and keep up with technological advancements to help positively influence diabetes care in the future.

CHAPTER 10

Living Proof: Heartwarming Narratives of Recovery

This chapter features heartwarming accounts of people who overcame type 2 diabetes by being determined, resilient, and committed to their health. These narratives illustrate the process of conquering obstacles, preserving sustainability over the long run, and sharing a message of hope with those who are experiencing comparable health issues.

10.1: Success Stories: Actual People Curing Their Diabetes

Maria's Road to Recovery

After years of battling weight gain and erratic blood sugar readings, 52-year-old Maria was finally diagnosed with type 2 diabetes. Maria sought advice from a healthcare team that specialized in managing diabetes, driven by her desire to take back control of her health.

Maria completely changed her eating habits by cutting back on processed sugars and carbohydrates and focusing on nutritious foods under the individualized advice of a dietician. She added regular walks to her schedule and progressively upped her physical activity level with yoga sessions. Maria's blood sugar returned to normal in six months, and she was able to stop using her diabetes medicine.

Maria keeps up her healthy lifestyle by eating a balanced diet, exercising frequently, and practicing yoga. Her achievement is attributed to the continuous assistance of her medical team and her determination to put her health first.

John's Journey to Well-Being

John, a 45-year-old IT specialist, was diagnosed with diabetes after experiencing extreme weariness and frequent thirst. This was a wake-up call for him. John started a journey of lifestyle change because he was determined to get healthier and stay off medicine.

He began by being knowledgeable about diabetes care and nutrition, learning how to interpret food labels and make wise decisions. John gradually increased his level of fitness by adding cardiovascular and strength training routines to his weekly routine. John started eating a low-carb diet full of veggies, lean meats, and healthy fats after receiving advice from a diabetic educator.

John's perseverance paid off in due course. His energy returned, his blood sugar regulated, and he shed some weight. John still places a high priority on his health now. He routinely checks his blood sugar levels, keeps himself active by going on walks and working out at the gym.

10.2: Meeting Difficulties Head-On and Solving Problems Along the Way

Overcoming a variety of obstacles that offer chances for development and fortitude is necessary to reverse type 2 diabetes:

Managing Social Environments

In social settings when poor eating choices were common, Maria and John both had difficulties. By making advance plans, packing wholesome foods, and sharing their health objectives with loved ones, they discovered how to successfully negotiate these situations.

Storage of Emotions

Maria suffered from emotional eating patterns brought on by job stress. She learned how to manage stress without turning to food by attending counseling sessions and support groups. Coping mechanisms she adopted included journaling and mindfulness exercises.

Acclimating to Shifts in Lifestyle

During his hectic work weeks, John found it difficult to stick to his fitness regimen. By planning workouts into his calendar and investigating adaptable fitness options including at-home workouts and lunchtime walks, he made physical activity a priority.

10.3: Sustainability over the Long Term - Sustaining a Healthful Lifestyle for Life

Sustainability is essential to long-term diabetes remission and general health:

Eternal Education and Adaptation

John and Maria both stress how crucial it is to keep learning and making adjustments as they pursue their health goals. To fine-tune their lifestyle choices, they attend diabetes education programs, remain up to date on new research, and routinely confer with their healthcare team.

Support and Community

Maria and John derived strength from their networks of support, which included local support groups, online diabetic communities, and close friends and family who served as sources of inspiration and encouragement during their journey.

10.4: A Hope-Filled Story: You Can Reverse Type 2 Diabetes and Govern Your Own Health

We can personally attest from Maria's and John's experiences that diabetes reversal is possible with dedication, knowledge, and assistance. Their stories demonstrate the value of a caring healthcare staff, the transformational effect of lifestyle modifications, and persistence.

Through the presentation of these motivational tales, useful suggestions, and an optimistic outlook, this chapter hopes to encourage readers to take charge of their health, adopt new lifestyle choices, and embark on a journey to reverse diabetes and achieve long-term wellbeing. Although every path is different, people can achieve amazing improvements in their health and quality of life with perseverance and assistance.

ABOUT THE AUTHOR

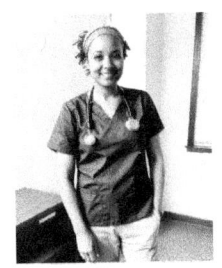 Harmony Royce is a dedicated healthcare worker who has a strong interest in holistic wellness. Harmony's extensive history in various aspects of health and wellness provides her with a wealth of knowledge and expertise that she can utilize in her writing and professional endeavors.

Harmony is a talented author who crafts thought-provoking books that inspire readers to have well-rounded, balanced lives. She writes about a variety of health-related topics, such as diet, exercise, mental health, and mindfulness. Her approachable writing style combines practical guidance with evidence-based research to make complex health concepts approachable and engaging for readers of all ages.

Harmony actively promotes the benefits of holistic health through writing, community workshops, and internet forums. Her mission is to educate and inspire people about the transformative power of self-care and healthy lifestyle choices.

www.ingramcontent.com/pod-product-compliance
Lightning Source LLC
Chambersburg PA
CBHW072053230526
45479CB00010B/852